Best Keto Dessert Recipes 2021

The healthiest and tastiest

desserts in Keto style

Sommario

INTRODUCTION

Welcome to the world of Keto sweets!

How can you stay in shape without rewarding yourself with good, juicy desserts?

In this book, I wanted to put my 50 favorite keto dessert recipes so you can wow your whole family and friends. Show off your fit physique while eating a delicious dessert.

Let's get started right away by baking these low-sugar protein desserts that are ideal for the whole family, so put on your apron and let's get started right away.

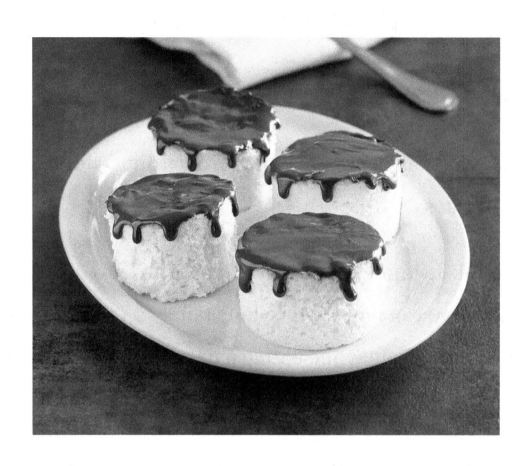

DESSERT RECIPES

CREAMY CHEESE WITH MACADAMIA AND PINEAPPLE CRUST

Ingredients

- 1 cup dried pine nuts

- 1 cup whole or half macadamia nuts

- 9 ½ Tbsp sucralose-based sweetener (sugar substitute)

- 3 Tbsp unsalted butter bar

- 16 g of cream cheese

- 3 large eggs (whole)

- 1 cup sour cream (cultivated)

- 1 Tbsp vanilla extract

- 2 lemon zest tsp

- ¼ tsp salt

Instructions

6. Preheat the oven to 350° F.

7. To make the crust: squeeze the nuts and 1 ½ Tbsp sugar substitute in a food processor until they are finely ground. Add the butter and mix to mix. With your fingers, gently press the nut mixture into the bottom of a fountain with 9 springs. Bake for 10 min and remove from the oven to cool.

8. To make the filling: Press the cream cheese and ½ cup sugar substitute in a food processor until smooth. Add eggs 1 by 1, squeeze well and scrape the bowl if necessary. Add sour cream, vanilla, lemon zest, and salt, and press to combine. For the filling into prepared crust.

9. Cook 40 min. Turn off the oven; Let the cheesecake cool for an hour without opening the door. Cool 12 to 24 hours. If desired, garnish with cranberries before serving.

Prep time:20 min **Servings:** 15

Macros: 7.2 g net Carbs 11.2 g protein 56.2 g fat 2.1 g fiber 569.8 Cal

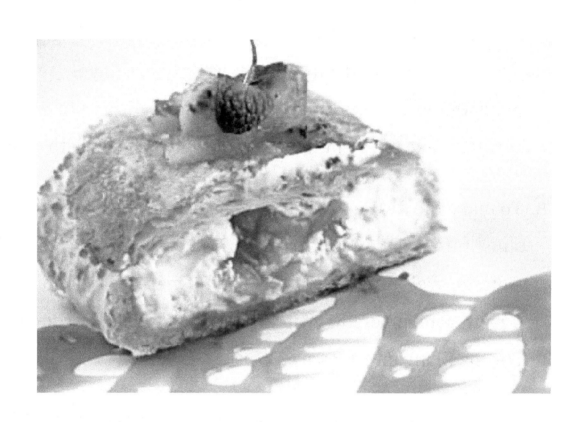

CREAMY CHOCOLATE SODA

Ingredients

- 4 Tbsp Hershey's unsweetened chocolate syrup

- 1 Tbsp heavy cream

- 1 can of Seltzer water

Instructions

1. Place ice cubes in a tall glass. Pour the sugar ingredients, then add the cream and 1 tsp chocolate extract or replace ½ tsp vanilla.

2. Fill the glass with mineral water and stir vigorously until mixture froths over the edge.

Prep time: 5 min **Servings:** 1

Macros: 4.4 g net Carbs 0.3 g protein 5.5 g fat 0 g fiber 71.4 Cal

BLACK MOCHA PUDDING

Ingredients

- 8 Servings: of organic coconut milk

- ½ cup heavy cream

- A pinch of salt

- ⅓ cup erythritol

- 3 tsp sucralose sweetener (sugar substitute)

- 2 large egg yolks

- 1 tsp dry coffee (instant powder)

- 1 Tbsp cocoa powder (sugar-free)

- ½ tsp Thick-It-Up

- 1 tsp vanilla extract

- ⅓ cup Lily's Sugar-Free Chocolate Chips

- 1 Tbsp unsalted butter

Instructions

7. Place 1 3/4 cups coconut milk in a saucepan with heavy cream, salt, and granulated sugar substitutes. Simmer over medium heat.

8. While the milk is heating up, beat the egg yolks with the remaining ¼ cup coconut milk and instant coffee. As soon as the milk mixture is hot, for a regular spray into the egg yolks while you beat. Once all of the milk has been absorbed, for the dough into the pan over medium heat. While warming up, quickly mix the cocoa powder and Thick-It-Up in a small bowl, then mix with the milk and egg mixture. Boil and stir the pudding continuously to prevent the egg from clotting. Boil until it begins to thicken (the mixture will still be slightly liquid); about 2-3 min Do not boil the pudding. Remove the heat as soon as it is thickened; about 3-5 min

9. Melt the chocolate with the butter in a small bowl in the microwave at 30-second intervals. Do not overheat to mix, then scrape the hot pudding while stirring to combine well. Keep away from heat.

10. Cool quickly on an ice-water bath; Place a plastic film on the surface to prevent skin formation. Once cool, place it in the refrigerator for additional cooling or immediately put it in bowls, cover with whipped cream if desired, and serve. Makes 2 2/3 cups. Each serving is ⅓ cup. This pudding is delicious, remember to serve it in a small glass dish with whipped cream.

Prep time: 10 min **Servings:** 10

Macros: 5.5 g net Carbs 2.6 g protein 22.4 g fat 0.8 g fiber 227 Cal

DECADENT CHOCOLATE CAKE

Ingredients

- Bake 4 g of sugar-free chocolate squares

- ½ cup unsalted butter bar

- 1 Tbsp tap water

- 3/4 cup sweetener based on sucralose (sugar substitute)

- 2 cocoa powder Tbsp (sugar-free)

- 1 tsp vanilla extract

- 6 large eggs (whole)

Instructions

1. Heat the oven to 325° F. Grease an 8-inch springform and cover the bottom with parchment paper; grease the paper and set aside.

2. Melt the chocolate, butter, and water over a double boiler over low heat, stirring to combine. Remove from heat and transfer to a large bowl; cool to room temperature. Add ¼

cup sugar substitute, cocoa powder, and vanilla extract to the chocolate mixture, stirring until well combined.

3. In a medium bowl, with an electric mixer on medium heat, beat the eggs until the mixture forms thick ribbons when the mixer is lifted, about 6 min. Reduce speed to average; Gradually add the remaining ½ cup sugar substitute and beat until combined, 1 minute. Stir in a third of the egg mixture into the chocolate mixture to make it lighter. In 2 additions, fold the rest of the egg mixture until it is well mixed.

4. Pour the dough into prepared pan and smooth the top. Bake in the oven until evenly raised and almost done, 40 to 45 min (it looks like a brownie). Let cool entirely on a wire rack. Stick a knife along the edge of the pan and remove the side to serve. Cut into 12 pieces and serve with whipped cream (optional).

Prep time: 15 min **Servings:** 12

Macros: 3.1 g net Carbs 4.7 g protein 14.9 g fat 1.6 g fiber 159.3 Cal

DECADENT CHOCOLATE ICE CREAM

Ingredients

- 3 cups heavy cream

- 2 large egg yolks

- 4 large eggs (whole)

- 3/4 cup cocoa powder (sugar-free)

- 3/4 cup sweetener based on sucralose (sugar substitute)

- ¼ tsp salt

- 2 tsp vanilla extract

- ½ tsp pure almond extract

Instructions

1. Pour the heavy cream into a 3-liter thick-bottomed saucepan and place over medium heat. Simmer, but do not cook. Remove from heat and set aside.

2. Combine eggs, yolks, cocoa powder, sugar substitute, and salt in a large bowl. Beat with an electric mixer in the middle until it is thicker and smoother, 2 to 3 min, scrape the sides of the bowl with a rubber spatula. Remove a cup of hot cream from the pan with a ladle and gradually mix in the egg mixture (this will temper the eggs, so they don't curdle). While beating, for the hot egg mixture into the rest of the cream in a saucepan.

3. Place over medium heat and beat until slightly thicker and cover the back of a wooden spoon; the temperature should not exceed 170° F.

4. Pour into a clean container, mix the extracts and let stand until the cream has cooled to room temperature, about 1 ½ hours, or place it in a neat box set in a larger container filled with a water bath. Let cool for 2 hours or cover with plastic wrap and let refrigerate overnight to develop more flavor.

5. Freeze in the ice-cream maker according to the manufacturer's instructions. When the freezing process is complete, serve immediately for soft or firm ice, place in an airtight container and freeze for 2-4 hours or overnight. (It

can be stored in the freezer for up to 1 month). It is about 1 liter, each serving = ½ cup.

Prep time: 25 min **Servings:** 8

Macros: 6.7 g net Carbs 7.2 g protein 37.7 g fat 2.7 g fiber 388.5 Cal

BERRY POPSICLES

Ingredients

- 2 cups unroasted blueberries (sugar-free, frozen)

- 3/4 cup tap water

- 4 Servings: of unsweetened strawberry syrup

- 1 tsp orange zest

Instructions

1. Process the blueberries, water, sugar and zest in a blender until smooth.

2. Pour into plastic molds to make ice and freeze for about 3 hours. NOTE: 4 Servings: of syrup equals ½ cup.

Prep time: 5 min **Servings:** 4

Macros: 4.9 g net Carbs 0.2 g protein 0.3 g fat 1.4 g fiber 33.2 Cal

DOUBLE CHOCOLATE COOKIES

Ingredients

- ¼ cup unsalted butter bar

- ¼ cup xylitol

- 1 tsp vanilla extract

- 1 large egg (whole)

- 1 ½ cups blanched almond flour

- 2 cocoa powder Tbsp (sugar-free)

- ¼ tsp baking powder

- ¼ tsp salt

- 3 packets of Endulge chocolate candies

Instructions

1. This is suitable for all phases except for the first 2 weeks of nut induction. 1 cookie = 1 serving.

2. Preheat an oven to 350° F. Use a Silpat mat or baking paper on the baking sheet.

3. Beat the soft butter with xylitol until it is smooth and fluffy; about 3 min Add vanilla and egg and beat until everything is well combined.

4. Combine all remaining dry ingredients, except candy, stir to mix, then add to wet ingredients. Mix until completely absorbed, then add the candy.

5. Form balls of 18 x 1 inch, spaced 1 inch apart, and flatten them slightly on the baking sheet. Bake for 10 min, remove from the oven and let stand for 5 min, then move it to a cooling rack. Cookies can be stored for up to 2 days in an airtight container at room temperature.

Prep time:10 min **Servings:** 6

Macros: 1.3 g net Carbs 2.7 g protein 8.7 g fat 1.9 g fiber 107.1 Cal

DOUBLE CHOCOLATE WALNUT ICE CREAM

Ingredients

- 1 cup chopped nuts

- 1 tsp gelatin powder

- 1 cup tap water

- 6 large egg yolks

- 3/4 cup sweetener based on sucralose (sugar substitute)

- 2 ½ cups heavy cream

- 2/3 cup cocoa powder (sugar-free)

- ½ tsp salt

- 1 ½ tsp vanilla extract

- 4 Tbsp Lily's sugar-free chocolate chips

Instructions

1. Preheat to 350° F.

2. Roast the nuts for 8 min, remove and let cool, then chop and set aside. Sprinkle gelatin over water in a thick-bottomed pot. Let sit until soft, about 5 min

3. In a medium bowl, beat the yolks and sugar substitute to combine. Add the cream and cocoa powder to the gelatin mixture and cook over medium heat, occasionally stirring, until the cocoa dissolves and the mixture begins to simmer.

4. Slowly for half of the gelatin mixture into the yolk mixture and beat consistently. Return the mixture to the pot. This process is called quenching. Cook, constantly stirring, until mixture is thick enough to cover the back of a spoon, about 4 min Keep away from heat.

5. Add salt, vanilla and chocolate extracts. Cool the mixture for 4 hours. For the ice into the refrigerator. Treat according to the manufacturer's instructions. Add the nuts and chocolate about 5 min before the ice cream is ready.

Prep time:30 min **Servings:** 12

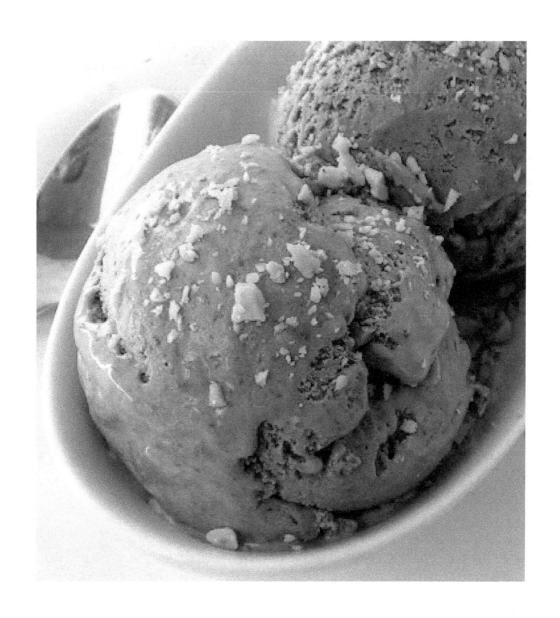

CHOCOLATE DOUBLE Protein PANCAKES

Ingredients

- ½ cup ricotta cheese, whole milk

- 2 each egg

- 29 g of protein powdered milk chocolate

- ¼ tsp baking powder

- ½ tsp ground cinnamon

- A pinch of salt

- 2 Tbsp Lily's sugar-free chocolate chips

- 1 ⅓ Tbsp coconut oil

Instructions

9. Beat the ricotta cheese and the eggs.

10. Add the protein powder, baking powder, cinnamon, and salt. Mix with a uniform.

11. Heat 1 tsp oil in a nonstick skillet over medium-high heat. Once the pan is hot, add ¼ of the dough and smooth it into a 6-inch round shape with the back of a spoon. Sprinkle ¼ of the chocolate chips over the surface. Cook until bubbles begin to form in the pancake, then gently turn it over; Cook 2 to 3 min on each side. Repeat for the remaining dough to make 3 more pancakes.

12. These are delicious served with fresh berries, the syrup is not necessary as these pancakes are sweet in themselves. Each serving consists of 2 6-inch pancakes.

Prep time: 5 min **Servings:** 2

Macros: 7g Net Carbs 24.7g Protein 36.8g Fat 5.8g Fiber 461 Cal

ALMOND BUTTER TRUFFLE

Ingredients

- 6 Tbsp almond butter

- ½ cup canned coconut cream

- 29 g of protein powdered milk chocolate

- 1 pinch of salt

- 6 Tbsp chocolate chips, sugar-free

- ⅓ Tbsp coconut oil

Instructions

1. Combine almond butter, coconut cream, and salt in a medium bowl until well combined. If the almond butter and coconut cream are firm or cold, you may need to heat them in the microwave (in a microwave-resistant container) or in a pan of steaming water (in a heat resistant container) to absorb them completely.

2. Add the protein powder and mix until all the dust has worked, and a smooth texture is created. The mixture is slightly oily.

3. Cover a baking sheet with parchment paper. Make 12 balls by picking up a spoonful of the almond butter mixture and using your hands to form a ball. Place the balls on a baking sheet covered with parchment paper and place them in the freezer to cool 30 min

4. While the balls are cooling, use a double boiler (or in a medium heat resistant bowl over a saucepan with about 1 inch boiling water) to melt the chocolate chips and coconut oil, stirring until they soften entirely and have a uniform texture. Stay warm until the balls are cold.

5. Remove the balls from the freezer and roll the melted chocolate 1 by 1 to cover. Place each coated truffle again on parchment paper and place it in the refrigerator until the chocolate has hardened about 10 min Store in an airtight container in the fridge for up to a week.

Prep time: 55 min; **Servings:** 12

Macros: 1.8 g net Carbs 3.4 g protein 8.4 g fat 2.7 g fiber 94.6 Cal

CHOCOLATE AND AVOCADO MOUSSE

Ingredients

- 3 any California lawyer

- ½ cup unsweetened coconut milk

- ½ cup unsweetened chocolate chips

- 2 ½ Tbsp cocoa powder

- 2 Tbsp erythritol

- 3 tsp (3.5 g) Truvia

- 2 tsp vanilla extract

- A pinch of salt

Instructions

4. Crush the avocado and put it in a blender with the coconut milk. Mix until smooth.

5. While the avocados are mixed, place the chocolate chips in a microwave-safe bowl and heat for 20 seconds, mix well and

heat at 10-second intervals until it melts, stirring in the middle. Once melted, add it to the avocado mixture and continue mixing while scraping the sides.

6. Add cocoa powder, erythritol, Truvia, vanilla, and salt. Mix and scrape the sides until all the ingredients are well combined, and the foam is smooth and creamy. Add an additional ¼ tsp Truvia at a time if you want a softer foam.

Prep time: 10 min; **Servings:** 4

Macros: 5.5 g Net Carbs 5.2 g Protein 30 g Fat 12.1 g Fiber 375.9 Cal

GANACHE WITH CHOCOLATE BERRIES

Ingredients

- 8 g of strawberries

- 2 cups red raspberries

- 2 cups fresh blueberries

- 8 g unsweetened chocolate chips

- ⅓ cup heavy cream

- ½ tsp vanilla extract

Instructions

1. Mix the fruit and place it in 6 dessert bowls.

2. Heat the chocolate and cream in a small saucepan over low heat until they melt (this can be done in the microwave 30 seconds straight. Be careful not to overheat and burn the chocolate). Add the vanilla and stir until smooth.

3. Let cool slightly and sprinkle the sauce over the fruit just before serving.

Prep time: 10 min; **Servings:** 6

Macros: 9.5 g net Carbs 4 g protein 17.6 g fat 8.1 g fiber 286.3 Cal Cal

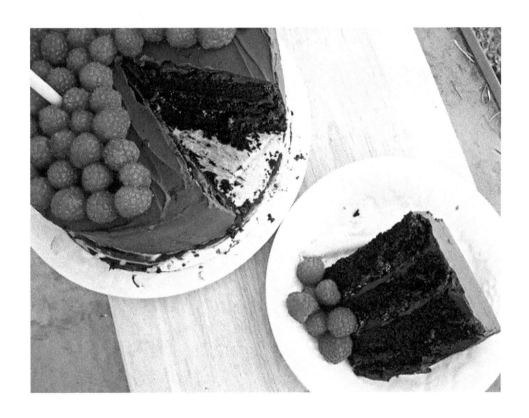

SWEET AND SOUR CHOCOLATE BROWNIES

Ingredients

- 2 Tbsp whole grain puff pastry

- 2 Tbsp whole-grain soy flour

- ¼ tsp baking powder

- 3 oz squares of baking chocolate without sugar

- 6 Tbsp heavy cream

- 2 Tbsp unsalted butter bar

- 2 large eggs (whole)

- 3/4 cup sucralose sweetener

Instructions

3. Preheat the oven to 375° F. Cover a baking sheet with parchment paper or aluminum foil.

4. In a large bowl, beat 2 Tbsp flour, soy flour, and baking powder.

5. In a microwave-safe bowl, melt the chocolate, cream, and butter for 1 to 2 min, until the butter melts and the chocolate is tender. Leave to stand for 2 min and stir until smooth. You can also perform this step on the stove.

6. Beat eggs and sugar substitute with an electric mixer on medium speed until soft and fluffy, about 3 min Gradually add the slightly hot chocolate mixture to the egg mixture until it is well combined, about 1 minute. Reduce the blender speed to low and mix the flour mixture that you have just combined.

7. Place slightly rounded tsp dough on the prepared sheet. Bake for 5 to 6 min, until done, but still soft on top. Put in a rack to cool completely.

Prep time: 15 min; **Servings:** 12

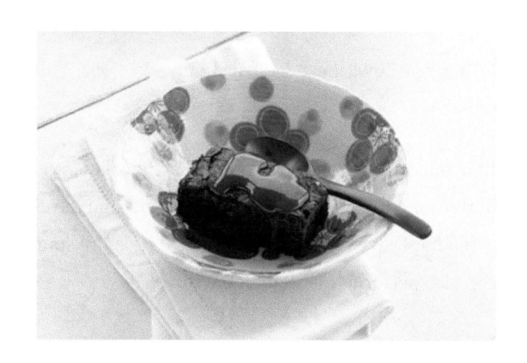

BLACKBERRY CLAFOUTI

Ingredients

- 6 g of blackberries

- 4 large eggs (whole)

- ⅓ cup xylitol

- 1/16 pinch of Stevia

- ¼ tsp salt

- ½ cup almond flour

- 1 cup heavy cream

- ¼ cup unsalted butter bar

- 1 tsp vanilla extract

- ½ tsp pure almond extract

- 1 tsp lemon zest

- ½ cinnamon tsp

Instructions

1. Preheat the oven to 325° F. Grease a shallow baking dish with butter. Place the blackberries in the baking dish and set aside.

2. Beat the eggs, granulated sugar substitutes, salt, and almond flour. Add the cream, ¼ cup melted butter, 1 tsp vanilla, ½ tsp almond extract, 1 tsp lemon zest (optional) and ground cinnamon; beat to combine.

3. For this mixture over the blackberries. Bake 35 to 45 min until puffed, golden, and placed in the middle. Let cool 20 min then serve hot or in the refrigerator for 3 days.

Prep time: 10 min; **Servings:** 8

Macros: 2.6 g net Carbs 5.3 g protein 22 g fat 1.8 g fiber 253 Cal

BLACKBERRY AND ORANGE SORBET

Ingredients

- 2 ¼ cups blackberries

- 1 orange zest tsp

- 1 cup buttermilk (less fat, cultivated)

- ⅓ cup sucralose sweetener

Instructions

1. Cook the blackberries, sugar substitute, 2 Tbsp water, and orange zest in a medium saucepan. Reduce the heat and simmer for 15 min, occasionally stirring, until the berries break. Cool quickly by placing it in a bowl located in another more giant bowl filled with an ice water bath.

2. Place the cooled berry mixture in a food processor. Transform into a smooth dough. Press through a fine colander into a bowl. Let cool in the refrigerator for 1 hour or until it is cold.

3. Pour into an ice maker and walk according to the manufacturer's instructions. Put in a bowl and freeze 2 to 3 hours before serving. 1 serving is equivalent to about ½ cup.

Prep time: 20 min; **Servings:** 4

Macros: 8.5 g net Carbs 3.6 g protein 1.6 g lipids 4.3 g fiber 75.9 Cal

RASPBERRY ALMOND CUPCAKES

Ingredients

- 2 large eggs (whole)

- 6 Tbsp Splenda sucralose sweetener, granulated

- ¼ cup unsalted butter bar

- 2 Tbsp heavy cream

- 1 our liquid tap water

- ½ tsp fresh lemon juice

- 1 tsp vanilla extract

- 2 tsp pure almond extract

- 1 ½ cups natural bleached almond flour

- ½ tsp baking powder

- ½ tsp salt

- 2 2/3 Tbsp jam

- canned red raspberries

Instructions

1. For best results, bring eggs and butter to room temperature.

2. Preheat the oven to 350° F. Place 8 paper molds in the form of muffins and set aside.

3. Separate the eggs and let the yolks separate. Beat the egg whites in a small bowl until they are frothy. Add 2 Tbsp sucralose and continue beating until stiff peaks form.

4. In another bowl, combine the butter and ¼ cup sucralose. Add the egg yolks, beating until they are well combined and light yellow. Slowly add cream, water, lemon juice, and extracts and beat until well blended. Carefully fold the egg whites into the egg yolk mixture.

5. Combine almond flour, baking powder, and salt in another bowl. Stir in the egg mixture carefully. Take about 2 Tbsp thick batter in each muffin pan. Use the back of a spoon to accurately make a small well and place 1 tsp raspberry jam in the middle.

6. Bake for 20 to 30 min until a stick in the middle comes out clean. Let cool in the pan for 20 min Enjoy hot or at room temperature. Keep the remaining cupcakes in an airtight container for up to a week and serve at room temperature. These can also be frozen for up to 1 month.

Prep time:15 min; **Servings:** 7

Macros: 5.1 g Net Carbs 7.1 g Protein 21.6 g Fat 2.6 g Fiber 242.5 Cal

APRICOT AND APPLE CLOUD

Ingredients

- 1 ½ cups heavy cream

- 2 Tbsp sucralose sweetener

- 16 g of applesauce and apricots for baby food

Instructions

1. Beat the cream and sugar substitute in the middle with an electric mixer until medium-firm peaks form.

2. Carefully fold in baby food (you need 16 oz or 4 oz jar oven).

3. Divide among 6 dessert bowls and let cool for at least 1 hour before serving.

Prep time:5 min; **Servings:** 6

Macros: 9.8 g net Carbs 1.4 g Protein 22.2 g Fat 1.4 g Fiber 241.7 Cal

DARK CHOCOLATE

Ingredients

- 1 cup heavy cream

- ½ cup tap water

- 2 cocoa powder Tbsp (sugar-free)

- ½ cup unsweetened chocolate syrup

- 1 tsp vanilla extract

Instructions

- In a medium saucepan, combine the cream, water, cocoa powder, and ½ cup unsweetened chocolate syrup.

- Bring to medium heat. Lower the temperature; Cook, occasionally stirring, for 5 min Remove from heat and add vanilla.

- For the mixture into 2 ice cube trays. Freeze 2 hours.

- Transfer the cubes to a food processor before serving. Press until the mixture is finely chopped and muddy.

Prep time: 5 min; **Servings:** 4

Macros: 6.4 g net Carbs 2.8 g protein 22.4 g fat 1.9 g fiber 229.5 Cal Cal

CINNAMON CAKE

Ingredients

- ¼ tsp salt

- 1 tsp sucralose sweetener (sugar substitute)

- 1 tsp cinnamon

- ½ cup unsalted butter bar

- 2 tap water Tbsp

- 3 3/4 portions, flour mixture

Instructions

1. Use the to make the flour mixture. You need 1 ¼ cups to make a pie crust.

2. Squeeze the pastry mixture, salt, sugar substitute, and cinnamon in a food processor to incorporate; add the butter and squeeze until mixture looks like a full meal, about 30 seconds. Press in the water until the dough collects, about 30 seconds (add 1 more Tbsp if necessary).

3. Transfer the dough to a plastic sheet; shape on a disc about 6 inches in diameter. Wrap well in plastic; Let cool to the firm, about 30 min

4. Roll and bake as directed in the cake . Makes 1 pie crust.

Prep time: 10 min; **Servings:** 4

Macros: 2.4 g net Carbs 9 g protein 13.5 g fat 1.6 g fiber 168.4 Cal

PANNA COTTA CARAMEL CAFÉ

Ingredients

- 1 sachet of gelatin, without sugar

- 2 Tbsp tap water

- 1 ½ cups heavy liquid cream

- 1 each, Caramel Shake Coffee

- 3 Tbsp erythritol (powder)

- 5 drops of liquid stevia

- 1 tsp vanilla extract

Instructions

1. Sprinkle the gelatin in a cup over the water and set aside.

2. Combine cream, smoothie, sweeteners, and vanilla in a small saucepan. Heat over medium heat, occasionally stirring, until it begins to simmer, about 10 min

3. Remove from heat and add gelatin until dissolved. Fill 6 molds with ½ cup liquid, cover with plastic wrap, and keep for at least 3 hours or until the gelatin is ready.

4. OPTIONAL: Serve with a Tbsp whipped cream

Prep time: 5 min; **Servings:** 6

Macros: 2.1 g net Carbs 4.7 g protein 23.5 g fat 0.2 g fiber 237.8 Cal Cal

NOEL BUCHE

Ingredients

- 8 eggs

- ½ cup Splenda

- 2 tsp vanilla extract

- 1 tsp espresso, instant powder

- A pinch of salt

- 4 Tbsp unsalted butter

- 8 Tbsp Lily's Sugar-Free Chocolate Chips

- 4 Tbsp cream, thick, liquid

- 5 cocoa powder Tbsp

- 3/4 tsp of baking powder

- 8 Servings: of Jello-o brand pudding without sugar or fat, chocolate

- 2 cups (8 fluid oz) of water

- 1 cup liquid (produces 2 cups of whipped cream)

- 1 cup unsalted butter

- 16 Tbsp cream cheese, original

- 3 Splenda packages

Instructions

1. Use instant coffee powder or instant coffee for this . For the frosting, you need 2 packs of sugar-free instant pudding.

2. Heat oven to 375° F. Butter the bottom and sides of an 11 x 17-inch pan. Separate the eggs by placing the Protein in a large bowl and set them aside.

3. For the cake: beat the 8 egg yolks and ½ cup sugar substitute (reserve 1 Tbsp to hit with the Protein in step 5) with an electric mixer on high speed, until ribbons compact form when the beaters (the pattern of the strip will appear after a few seconds in the dough). Add 1 tsp vanilla, espresso powder, salt, and soft butter and continue beating until smooth.

4. Melt chocolate and heavy cream in the microwave at 30-second intervals stir until completely melted and smooth. Add the egg yolks.

5. Sift cocoa powder and baking powder into a bowl. Add the egg mixture in 3 additions, beating after each addition. The dough will be thick and sticky. Put aside.

6. Beat the egg whites with clean whiskers and reserve 1 Tbsp sugar substitute with an electric mixer at high speed until firm peaks form. Add a third of the protein to the chocolate dough. Fold the remaining Protein in the mixture until they are completely absorbed. Roll out the dough in the prepared pans. Bake until done and a toothpick in the middle comes out clean, about 10 min Loosen the edges with a butter knife and let cool for 5 min

7. Turn the cake over on a large plastic covered plate. Place another piece of plastic on the cake. Start with a long edge and roll the cake to form a rod. Let cool on the baking sheet with the seam side down.

8. Empty the packaging of the pudding mixture into a large bowl for filling/frosting. Add water and beat until smooth.

Cool the pudding mixture and the whipped cream. In another bowl, beat the soft butter, soft cream cheese, and 1 Tbsp sugar substitute with an electric mixer on high temperature to obtain a smooth mixture. Pour the cold pudding into the butter mixture and beat on low speed until smooth. Add the whipped cream until smooth.

9. Roll the cake, remove the plastic wrap and spread about 3/4 of the filling on the surface, leaving a 1-inch border around it. Roll up the cake. (Remove excess material that drips from the edges and ends).

10. Make a diagonal cut through the cake about 3 inches from 1 end. Place the cut side of the short piece on top of the trunk to form the stump. Use the remaining frosting to freeze the outside of the cake and to smooth the edges where the log and stump meet and to freeze the sides of the stump and the ends of the stem.

11. Slide the teeth of a fork along the trunk to suggest the grain of the wood. Form concentric circles at the round end of the stump and at the terms of the log.

Prep time:35 min **Servings:** 18

Macros: 6.5 g net Carbs 5.3 g protein 27.6 g fat 4.1 g fiber 291.1 Cal

CRANBERRY ALMOND MOUSSE

Ingredients

- 4 Tbsp cream cheese, original

- 28 g vanilla protein powder

- 1 cup liquid (produces 2 cups of whipped cream)

- ⅓ tsp almond extract

- 1 cup fresh blueberries

- ¼ cup sliced almonds

Instructions

1. Mix the cream cheese and protein powder with an electric mixer until mixture is smooth. Put aside.

2. In another bowl, beat the heavy cream with the almond extract until it doubles in size.

3. Gently add ⅓ of the whipped cream to the cream cheese mixture until the mixture is smooth. Add another third of the whipped cream by folding it into the mixture until it is well

mixed. Add the 3rd end of the cream and fold until completely absorbed. Divide among 6 bowls, cover with plastic wrap and keep until ready to serve.

4. To roast the almonds, place them in a saucepan and roast for 3 to 5 min at 350° F. Sprinkle each bowl with cranberries and sliced almonds before serving.

Prep time: 15 min; **Servings:** 6

Macros: 5.1 g net Carbs 4.9 g protein 20.4 g fat 1.9 g fiber 222.7 Cal

BLACKBERRY AND PEACH COMPOTE

Ingredients

- 4 fluid oz Sauvignon Blanc wine

- 2 Tbsp xylitol

- 1 tsp ginger

- 1 tsp cinnamon

- 3 medium-sized peaches (2-1 / 2 "in diameter) (about 4 per lb)

- 6 g of blackberries

- ½ tsp Thick-It-Up

Instructions

1. Combine wine, granulated sugar substitute, ginger, ground cinnamon, and peaches in a medium pan. Bring to a boil, reduce the heat and simmer for about 15 min.

2. Add blackberries and Thick-It-Up; continue on low heat for 5 min

3. Remove from heat and allow to cool to room temperature or serve hot. It can be chilled for up to 1 week.

Prep time: 10 min; **Servings:** 12

Macros: 2.9 g net Carbs 0.4 g protein 0.1 g fat 3.3 g fiber 29.8 Cal

CARAMELIZED PEAR CAKE

Ingredients

- 2 Tbsp butter

- 2 Tbsp xylitol

- ¼ tsp ground cardamom

- 2 pears

- 3 large eggs (whole)

- 2 large egg yolks

- 2 cups heavy cream

- 2 Tbsp maple syrup (sugar-free)

- ½ oz liquid rum (without ice)

- 1 tsp vanilla extract

Instructions

1. Preheat the oven to 375° F.

2. Heat the butter, xylitol, and cardamom in a large skillet over medium heat. Cut the pears into ½ inch pieces. Once butter has melted, add the pears and caramelize for 4 min on each side. Remove from heat and place in a pie dish or 3-4 cup saucepan. Keep about 2 Tbsp syrup and pour the rest over the pears (keep the rest in the pan and set aside).

3. In a small bowl, beat the eggs, egg yolks, heavy cream, unsweetened syrup, rum, and vanilla in a combination. Pour mixture over pears and bake for 15-20 min until golden and the cream is hard. Remove from the oven and let cool slightly.

4. Brush the top with reserved caramel syrup with a pastry brush. When the sugar has hardened, heat it in the pan until it is liquid.

Prep time: 10 min; **Servings:** 8

Macros: 7.2 g net Carbs 4.4 g protein 27.9 g fat 1.3 g fiber 310.2 Cal

HAZELNUT BISCOTTI

Ingredients

- 1 ½ cups chopped hazelnuts

- 1 cup whole flour

- 1 tsp cinnamon

- ¼ tsp salt

- ¼ cup sour cream (grown)

- 4 large eggs (whole)

- 12 Tbsp unsalted butter

- 3/4 cup sucralose sweetener

- ⅓ cup dried cherries, sugar-free

Instructions

8. Heat the oven to 350° F.

9. Finely chop 1 cup hazelnuts (reserve ½ cup chopped hazelnuts). Place in a small bowl and mix with soy flour, ground cinnamon and salt. Combine sour cream and eggs in a medium bowl.

10. In a large bowl, with an electric mixer on medium speed, beat the butter with the sugar substitute for 3 min until it is creamy.

11. Add half of the egg mixture, beat for 30 seconds, and scrape the sides of the bowl with a spatula. Repeat this with the rest of the egg mixture. Turn on the mixer at low temperature and add dry ingredients, mix until they are combined. Fold the cherries and hazelnuts into large chopped pieces. Let the dough cool for 1 hour.

12. Divide the dough in half. On ungreased baking sheets, mold each half of the mixture on a 12 x 2½ inch wooden block. Cook the logs for 30 min, until they are almost firm. Transfer to a wire rack to cool for 10 min.

13. Lower the oven temperature to 325° F. Carefully cut the logs crosswise with a saw blade into ½ width slices. Place the

slices on baking sheets. Bake 17 to 20 min until firm and crisp. Cool the slices on baking sheets before storing them.

Prep time:45 min **Servings:** 10

Macros: 2.1 g net Carbs 2.4 g protein 7.5 g fat 0.8 g fiber 85.7 Cal

MINI CHOCOLATE LAYER PIES

Ingredients

- 2 ½ Tbsp Organic ground flax flour

- 2 tsp cocoa powder (sugar-free)

- A pinch of baking powder

- 1/16 tsp salt

- 1 oz Lily Sugar-Free Chocolate Chips

- 1 ½ Tbsp unsalted butter bar

- 1 Tbsp tap water

- 2 sour cream Tbsp (cultivated)

- 2 large eggs (whole)

- 1 tsp vanilla extract

- 3 Tbsp cream cheese

- 3/4 cup heavy cream

- 2/3 cup canned coconut cream

- 1 large yolk egg

- 2 Tbsp sucralose sweetener (sugar substitute)

- 6 Tbsp Torani sugar-free caramel flavor syrup

Instructions

For the pie

5. Preheat the oven to 350° F and set the grill to medium. Grease 6 wells of a muffin pan.

6. Combine flax flour, cocoa, baking powder, and salt in a small bowl; put aside.

7. Combine chocolate and butter in a medium-size microwave-proof bowl. Microwave in 30-second intervals, stirring at each interval until it melts; In total, about 3 min.

8. Beat the water, sour cream, ½ egg (beat an egg, divide the mixture in half, keep halFor the pie to add to the other berries), and ½ tsp vanilla. Add to the melted chocolate and stir until completely absorbed.

9. Add the flax mixture until it is combined. Spread the batter evenly over the 6 muffin trays.

Prep time: 20 min; **Servings:** 2

Macros: 3.9 g net Carbs 5.3 g protein 27.9 g fat 2.4 g fiber 283.9 Cal

CHOCOLATE PUDDING

Ingredients

- 1 serving, plus milkshake with creamy milk chocolate

- 3/4 cup heavy cream, liquid

- ¼ cup erythritol

- 1 Tbsp cocoa powder

- 1 ½ tsp xanthan gum

- 1 tsp vanilla extract

Instructions

1. Use a blender to combine all the ingredients until they are well combined and thick (about 30 seconds).

2. For a large amount of ½ cup pudding into 4 separate cups, cover with plastic wrap and let cool in the refrigerator for an hour before serving.

Prep time:2 min; **Servings:** 2

Macros: 2.2 g of net Carbs 8.7 g of protein 17.9 g oFat 2.2 g oFiber 207.5 Cal.

CHOCOLATE BUTTERCREAM

Ingredients

- ⅓ cup heavy cream

- 2 oz baked chocolate squares

- 8 Tbsp unsalted butter

- ½ tsp vanilla extract

- 1 Tbsp cocoa powder (sugar-free)

- 6 packets of calorie-free sweeteners

Instructions

1. Heat the cream in the microwave until it boils (about 1 minute).

2. Pour over the chopped chocolate in a small bowl.

3. In a large bowl, beat the butter and sugar substitute with an electric mixer.

4. Add the cocoa powder, chocolate and vanilla then add melted chocolate.

5. Keep whisking until it is soft and fluffy.

Prep time: 20 min; **Servings:** 4

Macros: 2.1 g net Carbs 1.4 g protein 19 g fat 1.4 g fiber 176.5 Cal

CHIA, CHOCOLATE AND COCONUT PUDDING

Ingredients

- 1 Generous Dark Chocolate Smoothie

- 4 Tbsp chia seeds

- ¼ cup coconut, grated, sugar-free

Instructions

1. In a medium-sized glass jar with a lid, mix all ingredients until well blended. Cover with a lid and leave in the refrigerator for at least 2 hours or overnight.

2. Cover with a pinch of cocoa beans), chopped almonds, or fresh whipped cream.

Prep time: 5 min; **Servings:** 2

Macros: 2.4 g of net Carbs 7.6 g of protein 12.2 g oFat 7.5 g oFiber 175.3 of Cal

CHOCOLATE AND MINT CHEESECAKE BARS

Ingredients

- Bake 2 g of sugar-free chocolate squares

- 2 ¼ cups heavy cream

- ¼ cup unsalted butter bar

- ½ cup erythritol

- 2 tsp vanilla extract

- 2 large eggs (whole)

- 1 ⅓ cup tap water

- 1 3/4 cups sucralose sweetener (sugar substitute)

- ¼ cup cocoa powder (sugar-free)

- 1 cup blanched almond flour

- 1 ½ tsp of baking powder (straight phosphate, double effect)

- ½ tsp salt

- 1 pack of powdered gelatin (sugar-free)

- 16 g of cream cheese

- A pinch of of mint extract (mint)

- 8 Tbsp Hershey Unsweetened Chocolate Syrup

Instructions

1. Use erythritol powder (you need about ½ cup granules to make 1 cup powder). It can easily be sprayed in a blender. Measure it after it is in powder form.

Bottom layer:

2. Preheat an oven to 350° F and grease a 9 x 13 x 2-inch nonstick skillet; put aside. Melt the chocolate and ¼ cup heavy cream in a small bowl in the microwave 20 seconds apart. Once melted, stir to combine and set aside to cool.

3. Beat the butter and 1 cup erythritol powder in a blender for 5 min until it is soft and fluffy. Add the vanilla and the mixed eggs 1 by 1 for 30 seconds between each egg. Add the cooled chocolate mixture and beat until well blended. Add ⅓ cup water and ½ cup sucralose, beat for 1 minute.

4. In a small bowl, combine cocoa powder, almond flour, baking powder, and salt. Add to the dough and mix for 1 minute until everything is thoroughly mixed. Pour batter into prepared pan and bake for 20 min or until a center stick comes out clean. Let cool. Prepare the top layer during cooling.

Top layer:

5. Add the gelatin packet to 1 cup boiling water. Mix until all the gelatin dissolves, then place in the refrigerator for about 10 min (do not allow to stand completely, only cool to room temperature).

6. Beat the cream cheese in a medium bowl with 1 cup sucralose until it is thoroughly mixed and smooth. Add the mint extract and enough green coloring to reach the desired color depth (about ¼ tsp). Once the gelatin has thoroughly cooled, mix it with the cheese mixture.

7. Beat the remaining 2 cups of cream with the remaining ¼ cup sucralose until semi-rigid peaks form. Gently fold the cream into the cheese mixture until it is completely absorbed. For this over the cooled brownie layer in the pan and leave in the refrigerator for 4 hours or overnight.

8. When they are ready to serve, cut them into 24 squares and cover with 1 tsp unsweetened chocolate syrup (Smucker's sugarless Sundae syrup works great because it is a little thicker than regular sugar). To make a spider web: start in the middle of the square to make a spiral. Take a toothpick and pull straight from the center to the outside edge. Repeat 5-6 times equally spaced.

Prep time: 20 min; **Servings:** 12

Macros: 4.7 g net Carbs 4.9 g protein 20.8 g lipids 1.1 g fiber 219.8 Cal

CHOCOLATE MINT MOUSSE

Ingredients

- 1 ½ cups heavy cream

- 1 Tbsp chocolate whey protein

- ¼ tsp mint extract

Instructions

1. Beat the cream with an electric mixer until thickened.

2. Add the protein mixture and ¼ to ½ tsp mint extract.

3. Keep beating until it is smooth and firm. Divide into bowls and let cool 30 min.

Prep time: 20 min; **Servings:** 5

Macros: 2.2 g net Carbs 13.7 g protein 22 g fat 0 g fiber 260.3 Cal

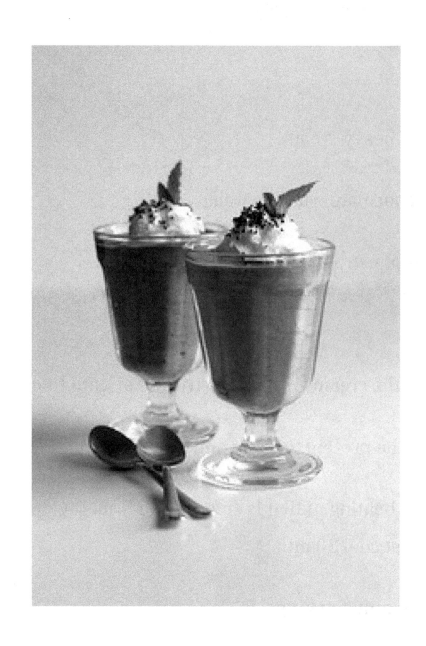

CHOCOLATE MOUSSE

Ingredients

- 7 g of unsweetened chocolate chips

- 1 ½ oz protein (dried)

- ½ cup tap water

- ¼ cup cocoa powder (sugar-free)

- 2 cups heavy cream

- 1 tsp dry coffee (instant powder)

- 1 tsp vanilla extract

- 2 Tbsp sucralose sweetener (sugar substitute)

Instructions

1. Melt the chocolate chips in a double kettle over medium heat (or in the microwave over medium heat for 1 to 2 min). Reserve and allow to cool to room temperature.

2. While the chocolate is cooling, beat 3 Tbsp dried white and water in a medium bowl with an electric mixer on medium speed, until the white is completely dissolved and firm peaks form about 5 min Put aside.

3. In a large bowl, combine cocoa powder with ½ cup cream, instant coffee, and vanilla until blended. Add the melted chocolate and set aside.

4. In another large bowl with an electric mixer, beat the remaining cream with a sugar substitute until semi-rigid peaks form for about 4 min Reserve 1 cup this sweet whipped cream (to cover) and incorporate the rest into the chocolate mixture in 2 additions.

5. Double the Protein in the chocolate cream mixture in 3 additions. Divide over 4 dessert glasses and cover with reserved whipped cream. Use a peeler to shave the remaining beautiful pieces of chocolate over the whipped cream if desired and serve.

Prep time: 15 min; **Servings:** 4

Macros: s 9.7 g net Carbs 15.6 g protein 60.5 g fat 5.3 g fiber 714.5 Cal.

MINI CHEESECAKES WITH CHOCOLATE MOUSSE

Ingredients

- 3 oz squares of baking chocolate without sugar

- 16 g of cream cheese

- ½ cup sucralose sweetener (sugar substitute)

- 3 large eggs (whole)

- 3/4 cup heavy cream

- 3/4 tsp pure almond extract

- ½ tsp vanilla extract

Instructions

1. Heat the oven to 325° F.

2. Heat the chocolate in the microwave in 30-second steps until it completely melts; cool slightly.

3. In a large bowl beat the cream cheese on medium speed. Add the chocolate and beat until smooth. Add sugar substitute and beat until everything is mixed.

4. Add eggs 1 by 1 and beat well after each addition. Add the cream and almond and vanilla extracts and beat until smooth.

5. For the mixture into prepared cream cups. Carefully for boiling water into the pan to roast half of the mussels.

6. Bake in the oven until cheesecakes are puffed, and centers are ready for about 20 min Remove from the oven and let stand in a water bath for 10 min

7. Transfer the custard cups to a wire rack; cool to room temperature. Cool to very cold, 4 hours or overnight.

8. Garnish with mint sprigs, chocolate chips, and raspberries, if desired.

Prep time: 10 min; **Servings:** 1

Macros: 5.2 g net Carbs 8.6 g protein 35.1 g fat 1.5 g fiber 362.5 Cal

CHOCOLATE MUDSLIDE

Ingredients

- 1 cup heavy cream

- 8 Tbsp Hershey Unsweetened Chocolate Syrup

- ½ cup tap water

- 3 Tbsp cocoa powder (sugar-free)

- 1 tsp vanilla extract

Instructions

1. Combine cream, ½ cup syrup, water, and cocoa powder in a medium saucepan.

2. Bring to medium heat.

3. Lower heat; Cook, occasionally stirring, for 5 min Remove from heat and add vanilla.

4. For the mixture into 2 ice cube trays. Freeze 2 hours.

5. Before serving, transfer the cubes to a food processor and mix until mixture is finely chopped and muddy.

6. Serve immediately.

Prep time:120 min

Macros: 7.6 g of net Carbs 2 g of protein 22.6 g oFat 1.3 g oFiber 232.6 Cal Cal

PEANUT BUTTER CHOCOLATE

Ingredients

- ½ cup Lily's Dark Chocolate Chips

- 2 Tbsp Lily's sugar-free chocolate chips

- 2 Tbsp peanut butter, creamy of course

- 3 drops of liquid stevia

- 1 pinch of salt

Instructions

7. Heat the dark chocolate chips for 30 seconds in a safe microwave bowl until they melt. Stir the chocolate and, if not completely melted, boil in the microwave at 10-second intervals and stop stirring between each until it is completely melted.

8. Bake the dark chocolate melted on a baking sheet covered with parchment in a uniform thin layer (1/8 inch thick).

9. Clean the microwave-safe container and heat the chocolate chips with milk in the microwave for 30 seconds or until it melts. Combine peanut butter, stevia drops and salt in melted milk chocolate chips in a combination.

10. Sprinkle the peanut butter mixture over the dark chocolate and use a skewer to shake the layers. Place in the refrigerator until it is firm, about 1 hour. Break into pieces and enjoy.

Prep time: 10 min; **Servings:** 2

Macros: 3.3 g net Carbs 3.9 g protein 12.4 g fat 8.3 g fiber 126.3 Cal

CHOCOLATE CHIP COOKIES WITH PEANUT BUTTER

Ingredients

- 3/4 cup whole flour

- 1 Tbsp cocoa powder (sugar-free)

- 3/4 cup sweetener based on sucralose (sugar substitute)

- ¼ tsp salt

- ⅓ cup natural creamy peanut butter ⅓ less sodium and sugar

- ½ cup heavy cream

- 2 large eggs (whole)

- 1 tsp vanilla extract

Instructions

1. Heat the oven to 375° F. Lightly spray baking sheets with an oil spray.

2. Beat soy flour, cocoa powder, sugar substitute, and salt in a bowl. In another bowl, combine the peanut butter, cream,

eggs, vanilla and chocolate extract (1 tsp; optional) until smooth. Add to dry ingredients; Stir until everything is mixed.

3. Place dough through Tbsp on greased baking sheets to form 18 cookies, 1 to 2 inches apart. Smooth the paste with your fingertips and flatten the cookies with a fork. Bake 8 to 10 min or until golden.

4. Let the cookies cool on the baking sheets for 1 minute before placing them on the racks so that they cool completely.

Prep time: 15 min; **Servings:** 4

Macros: 2.6 g net Carbs 3.6 g protein 6.5 g fat 0.9 g fiber 86.5 Cal

FROZEN BANANA BITES

Ingredients:

- A cup of peanut butter

- One-third cup of toffee baking bits

- One oz. of semisweet chocolate

- Four bananas (cut into rounds of one-inch thickness)

- One tbsp. of shortening

Instructions

1. First, take a wax paper and cover the baking sheet.

2. Then, take each slice of banana and layer with one spoon of peanut butter. Take a toothpick and insert it through the banana piercing through the layer of peanut butter. Then, take the banana bites and arrange them nicely on the baking sheet. Freeze the preparation for at least thirty minutes or overnight.

3. Now, melt the chocolate and keep stirring it frequently. To avoid any form of scorching, use a spatula to scrape down the sides continuously.

4. Take another waxed paper to cover another baking sheet.

5. Take two to four bites of bananas from the freezer at a time and then use the chocolate mixture to coat them. Now, take the coated bites and place them on this baking sheet that you just covered with wax paper. On top of each coated banana, sprinkle some toffee bits. Do the same process with all the bites. Now, return the preparation into the freezer and keep it there for at least an hour. Before serving, keep the bites at room temperature for around ten to fifteen minutes.

Preparation Time: 20 minutes **Servings:** 48 bites

Cooking Time: 2 hours 15 minutes

Nutrition: Calories: 76 Protein: 1.8gFat: 5.1g Carbs: 6.9gFiber: 1g

ITALIAN KALE CHIPS

Ingredients:

- Four cups of kale (stems removed, loosely torn)

- One-eighth tsp. each of

- Salt

- Pepper

- Garlic powder

- A quarter tsp. of Italian seasoning

- One tbsp. of olive oil

- Optional – One tbsp. of grated Parmesan cheese

Instructions

1. Set the temperature of the oven to 225 degrees Fahrenheit and preheat. The temperature of the oven is very important in this recipe; otherwise, your kale chips might just get burnt.

2. Now, it is time to prepare the kale. Tear the leaves and remove the stems. The leaves should be torn into bite-sized pieces.

3. Then, take a baking sheet and use cooking spray to coat it. After that, take the kale leaves and arrange them on the sheet in a single layer. Drizzle some more oil. Remember that too much oil can make the kale chips soggy, so be aware of how much oil you are using.

4. Now, take a small-sized bowl and in it, add garlic powder, Italian seasoning, pepper, and salt and mix them together. After mixing thoroughly, sprinkle this mixture evenly over the kale.

5. Once all of this is done, take the kale preparation and bake it for twelve minutes. After that, take them out, toss them a bit so that they get turned, and then return the preparation to the oven again. Bake for another five to ten minutes. By this time, the kale should be crispy. But keep a close eye on them since you don't want the burnt.

6. Once done, remove, and if you want, then sprinkle some grated Parmesan on top.

Preparation Time: 5 minutes **Servings:** 2 servings

Cooking Time: 15 minutes

Nutrition: Calories: 148 Protein: 6g Fat: 9g Carbs: 15g Fiber: 5g

APPLE AND QUINOA BARS

Ingredients:

- A quarter cup of peanut butter

- One cup each of

- Apple sauce (unsweetened)

- Coconut oil

- One tsp. of vanilla

- Half a tsp. each of

- Baking powder

- Cinnamon

- Two eggs

- One and a half cups each of

- Rolled oats

- Quinoa (cooked and cooled)

- One apple (chopped after peeling)

Instructions

1. Set the temperature of the oven to 350 degrees Fahrenheit and preheat.

2. Take a baking dish of 8 by 8 inches and coat it with oil. After that, keep it aside.

3. Take a large-sized bowl and add the peanut butter, apple sauce, eggs, coconut oil, cinnamon, and vanilla in it and mix them all together.

4. Now, take the cooked quinoa and mix it too along with the baking powder and rolled oats. Keep mixing until everything is properly incorporated.

5. Then, fold the apple in.

6. After that, scoop out the mixture and spread it on the prepared baking dish. Make sure that it has covered every corner evenly.

7. Bake the preparation for about forty minutes. After it is done, a toothpick inserted should come out without anything on it.

8. Before you slice or store it, the bars should have cooled completely.

Preparation Time: 30 minutes **Servings:** 12 servings

Cooking Time: 1 hour

Nutrition: Calories: 230Protein: 7g Fat: 10gCarbs: 31g Fiber: 4g

AVOCADO TOAST

Ingredients:

- One garlic clove

- Four slices of bread (whole wheat variety)

- One tsp. of parsley (finely chopped)

- Juice of half a lemon

- One avocado

- To taste – Pepper and salt

- For toppings – One tsp. of hemp seeds and some olive oil

Instructions

1. Start by toasting the sliced of bread and use a toaster to do so. You can also do it on the stove. Once you have toasted them based on your preference, remove and place them on the plates.

2. Take the avocado and slice it in half. First, remove the pit and then use a spoon to scoop out the flesh of the avocado. Take a small bowl and put the flesh in it. Then, season with pepper and salt and add the juice of half a lemon. Then, add the parsley.

3. Use a fork to make a creamy mash of the avocado mixture and make sure that all the ingredients have combined well.

4. Take the garlic clove and crush it with the help of a fork. Remove the peel and then take the inside of the garlic and rub it a bit on top of the toasts.

5. Then, scoop out the avocado mash you made and spread them evenly on the slices. If you want, you can sprinkle some hemp seeds on top and drizzle a bit of olive oil.

Preparation Time: 5 minutes **Servings:** 4 servings

Cooking Time: 5 minutes

Nutrition: Calories: 156.4 Protein: 5.1g Fat: 8g Carbs: 13.3g Fiber: 4g

TUNA PROTEIN BOX

Ingredients:

- Four carrots (chopped and peeled)

- Four whole eggs

- One cup of grapes

- Two to three celery ribs (chopped nicely)

- One cup of blueberries

- Eight ounces of cubed cheese

For the tuna salad:

- Two tbsps. each of

- Finely chopped celery

- Mayonnaise

- Five ounces of drained tuna

- Pepper and salt to taste

Instructions

1. Firstly, cook the eggs and make them hard-boiled. Leave them to cool and then peel them.

2. Take all the ingredients of the tuna salad and stir them all together. Once done, divide the preparation among all the four meal prep containers.

3. Take all the other ingredients as well and divide them among the containers.

4. You can refrigerate the meal for up to four days if you refrigerate.

Preparation Time: 10 minutes **Servings:** 4 servings

Cooking Time: 20 minutes

Nutrition: Calories: 414 Protein: 27g Fat: 25g Carbs: 20g Fiber: 3g

PUFFED QUINOA BARS

Ingredients:

- Three cups of quinoa (puffed)

- Half a cup each of

- Nut butter

- Packed soft dates

- Non-dairy milk

- A quarter cup of cacao powder

- Half a tsp. each of

- Sea salt

- Cinnamon

Instructions

1. Take a square baking pan of 8 inches and then use parchment paper to line it properly. Take a large-sized mixing bowl and place the quinoa in it.

2. Put the nut butter and dates in a food processor and blend on high. Blend it so that the mixture becomes completely smooth. Then, add cacao, milk, salt, and cinnamon. Pulse again until everything has blended properly.

3. Then, add this mixture of dates into the quinoa puffs and keep mixing to ensure everything has combined well. Then, take this mixture and press it into the baking pan that you lined. Press it so that it is as even as possible.

4. Now, take the baking pan and place it in the freezer for at least half an hour. Then take it out and refrigerate for two to three hours. After that, cut it into squares (approximately 16).

Preparation Time: 15 minutes **Servings:** 16 servings

Cooking Time: 40 minutes

Nutrition: Calories: 98 Protein: 3g Fat: 4g Carbs: 13g Fiber: 2g

ROASTED BROCCOLI

Ingredients:

- Five tablespoons of olive oil or coconut oil

- Three broccoli crowns (sliced into bite-sized florets)

- Two tablespoons each of

- Grated parmesan

- Lemon juice (freshly made)

- Four minced cloves of garlic

- Pepper to taste

Instructions

1. Set the temperature of the oven to 425 degrees Fahrenheit and preheat.

2. Prepare the florets of broccoli by slicing them into appropriate size and then place them all in a bowl.

3. Use coconut oil or olive oil to toss the broccoli florets along with pepper, salt, and garlic.

4. Now, arrange the broccoli evenly on a baking sheet.

5. Roast the preparation for about twenty to fifteen minutes.

6. Once done, remove the preparation from the oven and then sprinkle some parmesan cheese and lime juice on top.

Preparation Time: 15 minutes **Servings:** 6 servings

Cooking Time: 30 minutes

Nutrition: Calories: 211 Protein: 9g Fat: 12g Carbs: 21g Fiber: 7g

TUNA PATTIES

Ingredients:

- Ten oz. of tuna

- One tbsp. of dried chives

- One-third cup of panko or breadcrumbs

- Half a tbsp. of dried dill

- Two beaten eggs

- One tbsp. of Dijon mustard

- One tsp. of olive oil

- To taste – Pepper and salt

- Optional – lemon wedges

Instructions

1. Start by draining the tuna.

2. Then, take a large bowl and in it, add all the ingredients to mix them together.

3. Then, take the mixture to form four patties with your palm. Start by rolling then into balls and then shape them into patties.

4. Take a non-stick pan and heat the oil over medium flame. Add the patties and sauté them.

5. Cook each side of the patties for at least three to four minutes until they turn crisp and golden brown in color.

6. Take the lemon wedges and drizzle some juice on top of the patties.

Preparation Time: 5 minutes **Servings:** 2 servings

Cooking Time: 15 minutes

Nutrition: Calories: 249 Protein: 35g Fat: 8g Carbs: 8g Fiber: 1g

ROSEMARY KETO CRACKERS

Ingredients:

- ounces of almond flour

- Four tablespoons of hemp seeds

- One and two-thirds cup of parmesan cheese

- Half a teaspoon of onion powder

- Two tablespoons of rosemary (chopped)

- One ounce of butter

- Two large-sized eggs

- Half a teaspoon of salt

Instructions

1. Set the temperature of the oven to 375 degrees Fahrenheit and preheat.

2. In a mixing bowl, add all the dried ingredients. Whisk gently, but make sure that there are no lumps remaining.

3. Now, take a jug that is microwave-safe and place the butter in it. Melt the butter in the microwave. Add the eggs in this jug. Whisk the mixture until it becomes smooth.

4. Add this egg mixture onto the dry ingredients and mix thoroughly. A dough will form. At first, the dough can seem crumbly but keep pressing. Don't add any sort of liquids to the dough.

5. Keep the size of your over trays in mind and tear the baking paper accordingly. Now, take the dough and divide it in half. In case you are using smaller trays, divide it into quarters. Form the dough in the shape of a ball and place it on the baking paper.

6. Take another sheet and cover the dough. Use your rolling pin to press the dough. The layer should be around 3 millimeters. Once you have rolled them evenly, use a knife to form the shapes.

Preparation Time: 25min **Servings:** 20(5 crackers each)

Cooking Time: 50 minutes

Nutrition: Calories: 111 Protein: 5.9g Fat: 9.2g Carbs: 1.2g Fiber: 1g

CONCLUSION

We've come to the end of this trip, have you all baked?

I know at the beginning they may seem difficult to prepare but you just need to train a little bit, try and try again and you will see excellent results!

Dessert is always a meal very much appreciated by all, but that you can not always afford if you want to stay thin. Now you can.

I recommend everyone to always talk to a nutritionist before doing any diet, and enjoy the taste. Enjoy.

CPSIA information can be obtained
at www.ICGtesting.com
Printed in the USA
LVHW060318290321
682791LV00013B/1011